Baby Names

The Ultimate Book of Baby Names –
Includes the Latest Trends, Meanings,
Origins and Spiritual Significance

Jessica Ford

Table of Contents

Introduction **5**
Trending...**6**
   Boys 6
   Girls 10
   Unisex...14
Celtic **21**
   Boys 21
   Girls 23
   Unisex 25
Nordic **27**
   Boys 27
   Girls 29
   Unisex...31
German **33**
   Boys 33
   Girls 36
   Unisex...38
Historical **40**
   Boys 40
   Girls 42
   Unisex 44
Most Common **47**
   Boys 47
   Girls 51
   Unisex 56
Most Unusual **58**
   Boys 58
   Girls 60
   Unisex.. 63
Conclusion 71

Introduction

Congratulations on downloading your personal copy of *Baby Names: The Ultimate Book of Baby Names – Includes the Latest Trends, Meanings, Origins and Spiritual Significance.* Thank you for doing so.

The following chapters will provide you with lots of different baby names from around the world. Each chapter is broken down into boy, girl, and unisex names. Every name has information about what it means and where it originated along with many other interesting facts.

Picking your child's name is the first hardest decision you will have to make in your child's life, so why not have a little bit of help. This book has lots of names, and you are sure to find one that is perfect for your baby.

There are plenty of books on this subject on the market, thanks again for choosing this one! Every effort was made to ensure it is full of as much useful information as possible. Please enjoy!

Trending

Boys

Liam: The number one trending boy name is German. The Irish derivative of the German name *William* that contains the elements *wil* meaning 'desire' and *helm* meaning 'helmet' and together means 'strong-willed warrior'.

Noah: The number two trending boy name is of Hebrew origin and means 'comfort' or 'rest'. In the Old Testament, Noah built the Ark and saved his family and the animals from the Great Flood. He got a sign from God in the form of the rainbow. He fathered three sons Japheth, Ham, and Shem.

Elijah: The number three trending boy name is of Hebrew origin and means 'My God is Yahweh'. In the Old Testament, Elijah was a miracle worker and prophet. Elijah confronted King Ahab and Queen Jezebel over their worship of the idol Ba'al. He did not die but was carried to heaven in a chariot of fire. Since Elijah was popular in medieval tales, and the name was given by many saints, the name was regularly used during the middle ages. During medieval England, the name was spelled, *Elis*.

Logan: The fourth trending boy name is of Celtic origin. It was from the surname *Lagan* that was derived from a Scottish place name that means 'little hollow'.

Mason: The fifth trending boy name is of French origin. It is from the surname that is given to stone workers.

James: The sixth trending boy name is of Hebrew origin, and it means 'follower'. There were three James mentioned in the New Testament. *Saint James the Greater* was beheaded under Herod Agrippa. *James the Lesser* was the son of Alphaeus. *James the Just* was the brother of Jesus. The name has been used in England since the 1400s. It is more common in Scotland since it has seen several kings named James.

Aiden: The seventh trending boy name is of Celtic origin and means 'little fire'. It is an anglicized form of *Aodhan*. In the last part of the 1900s, it has risen in popularity in the US because of the sound *aden*.

Ethan: The eighth trending boy name is of Hebrew origin meaning 'firm', 'enduring', 'solid', or 'strong'. In the Old Testament, there weren't many characters with this name; the most notable is *Ethan the Ezrahite*. He was the writer of Psalm 89. It was used after the Protestant Reformation in the

English-speaking world. It got popular in America because of *Ethan Allen (1738-1789)*.

Lucas: The ninth trending boy name is of Latin origin and means 'light'. It is a variation of the Biblical name Luke. It is an English form of a Greek name meaning from Lucania. In the Bible, Luke was a physician that traveled with the Apostle Paul. He is thought to have been of Greek descent.

Michael: The tenth trending boy name is of Hebrew origin that means who is like God? Michael was one of the seven archangels. In the Old Testament in the book of Daniel, he is named as the protector of Israel. In Revelation, he is portrayed as heaven's army's leader. He is considered the patron saint of soldiers.

William: The next trending boy name is of German origin. It is derived from the elements *wil* meaning 'desire' or will and *helm* meaning 'protection' or 'helmet'. It is a variation of the name *Willahelm*.

Sebastian: The next trending boy name is of Latin origin. It is a version of the name *Sebastianus* which means 'from *Sebaste'*. This is a town in Asia Minor. Its name comes from the Greek *sebastos* meaning 'venerable'. Saint Sebastian was a Roman soldier that was martyred. When it was discovered he was a Christian, he was tied and shot with arrows. This didn't kill him.

Joseph: The next trending boy name is of Hebrew origin. It is from the Greek word *Ioseph* which is from the Hebrew name *Yosef* which means 'he will add'. In the Old Testament Joseph is a son of Jacob and husband to Rachel. He was his father's favorite and his brothers sold him into slavery. While in Egypt, Joseph gained fame and became an advisor to the pharaoh.

David: The next trending boy name is of Hebrew origin. It is derived from *Dawid* that was derived from *dwd* meaning 'beloved'. David was one of the greatest kings of Israel and ruled in the 900s BC. The most famous story is when he defeated Goliath, a huge Philistine. Jesus is said to be a descendant of him.

Gabriel: The next trending boy name is of Hebrew origin. It is derived from the Hebrew *Gavri'el*, meaning 'God is my strong man'. It could also be derived from *ever* which means 'hero or strong man'. Gabriel is an archangel and appears as God's messenger. In the Old Testament, he was sent to help Daniel interpret dreams. In the New Testament, he was sent to announce the birth of John and Jesus.

Girls

Emma: The number one trending girl name is of Latin origin. It was originally short for any Germanic name that began with the element *ermen* that means 'universal or whole'. Emma of Normandy was the wife of King Ethelred II and King Canute. She introduced the name to England. It also is derived by an Austrian saint that was called *Hemma*.

Olivia: The second trending girl name was popularized by Shakespeare. It was spelled this way by William Shakespeare in the comedy, Twelfth Night. Olivia is a wealthy, pampered Countess. In ancient Greece, this name meant 'olive' and was symbolic for Athena. It was also a token of fertility and peace. Olive wreaths were given as awards at the Olympic Games.

Ava: The third most trending name is from different origins. It has roots in German, Persian, and English. This name originally was a short form of German names that began with the element *avi* that probably meant 'desired'. In Persia, the name means 'sound or voice'. In the English origin, it is a variation of Eve.

Isabella: The fourth trending name of Hebrew origin. It is the Latin form of Isabel. It is a variation of Elizabeth that means 'devoted to God'. This name was held by many medieval royals like queen consorts of Hungary, Holy Roman Empire, Portugal, France, and England. And the powerful Queen Isabella of Castile.

Sophia: The fifth trending name is of Greek origin and means wisdom. This name comes from an early possibly mythical saint that died from grief after her daughters were slain during Emperor Hadrian's reign. Legends arose due to the misunderstanding of the phrase *Hagia Sophia,* meaning 'Holy Wisdom'. This is the name of the basilica in Constantinople. This name was common with royalty during the Middle Ages and became popular in Britain by the German Hanover House when they gained control of the throne in the 1900s.

Mia: The sixth trending name has German, Dutch, and Scandinavian roots. It is a derivative of Maria. It matches with the Italian word *mia* that means 'mine'. It is the Israeli abbreviation of *Michal.* In Latin, it means 'wished for child, bitter, or rebellion'.

Charlotte: The seventh trending name is of French origin, and it means 'free'. It is the feminine form of Charles and shares nicknames of Charley or Charlie. Other nicknames are Char, Lotta, and Lottie. Carlotta is the Italian form of Charlotte.

Amelia: The eighth trending name is of Hebrew origin. The Germanic spelling *Amalia* means 'work'. It could also be a variant of *Emilia* meaning 'rival'. In Latin, it means 'striving and industrious'. The Teutonic meaning is 'defender'.

Abigail: The ninth trending name is of Hebrew origin *Avigayil* meaning 'my father is joy'. When used as an English name, Abigail became common after the Protestant Reformation. It was popular with the Puritans, too. In the Old Testament, Abigail was Nabal's wife. After he died, she became King David's third wife. Abigail called herself a servant. In the 1600s the name was slang for servant. The name was not fashionable after that but was revived in the 1900s.

Emily: The tenth trending name is of Latin origin and means 'eager or striving'. It is an English cognate of the Latin name *Aemilia*, which derives from *Aemilius* that is an Old Roman family name that is derived from *Aemulus* meaning 'trying to equal or excel, rival'. The name Emily means 'strong, pretty, simple, classic, and feminine'.

Camila: The next trending girl name is of Portuguese and Spanish origin. It is a variation of *Camilla*. *Camilla* is the feminine of *Camillus*. This name is a legendary warrior maiden of the Volsci. *Camillus* goes back to Ancient Roman and its meaning is unknown. It may have been related to

Latin *camillus* meaning 'a youth employed in religious services'.

Ella: The next trending girl name is of French origin. It's a form of the name *Alienor*. She was called *Aenor* by her mother and was called *Alia Aenor* which means 'the other Aenor' by the Occitan. It is also short for *Eleanor*.

Zoey: The next trending girl name is of Greek, Italian, and English origins. It means 'life' in Greek. It was adopted by Jews as a translation of Eve. Zoe has been used since the 1800s. It is more common with Christians and has many different spellings.

Penelope: The next trending girl name is of English and Greek mythology origins. It is derived from the Greek *penelops,* a type of duck. It also has the elements of *pene* meaning 'weft or threads' and *ops* meaning 'eye or face'. It was the name of Odysseus's wife in Homer's epic poem 'Odyssey'.

Mila: The next trending girl name is of Slavic origin. It has the elements *milu* meaning 'dear and gracious.' In Slavic, it means 'hard working or industrious'. In Russia, it means 'dear one'. It is a pet form of the names Miloslava, Camila, Ludmila, Milica, Milan, and Milena. It has been connected to the Spanish name *Milagros* that means 'miracles'.

Unisex

Addison: This unisex name is of Hebrew origin and began life as an English surname, which means 'son of Adam'. It is also a Scottish patronymic surname that 'means son of Addie'. In the Scottish Lowlands, it is a nickname for Adam.

Ash: This unisex name is of Hebrew origin and began life as an English place-name. The Hebrew meaning is 'happy'. The English meaning is 'ash tree'. This name was derived from the element *Æsc* meaning 'ash tree' and *tun* which means 'enclosure, village, settlement, or town'.

Aubrey: This unisex name has roots in France and means 'ruler of elves or supernatural being'. It is an English given name. It is a Norman French version of the German given name *Alberic*. The name was derived from the element *alf or elf* and *ric* which means 'power'.

Bailey: This unisex name has roots in Middle English that referred to someone in the position of steward or official, bailiff, warrant officer. It is a topographical name for a person who resided near the outer wall of a castle. The name was derived from the Old English, *beg,* meaning 'berry' plus *leah* meaning 'woodland clearing'.

Bobbie: This unisex name is of German origin and means 'shining, bright, famed'. This name was introduced to the English by the Normans. In England, it is slang for policeman. Short for Robert which is derived from Old German *Hrodebert* with the elements *hruod* meaning 'fame' and *behrt* meaning 'bright'.

Brett: This unisex name is from the Celtic origin meaning 'a Breton'. In the English origin, it means a native of Brittany.

Brook: This unisex name has mixed origins of Old English and Old German. It means 'small stream'.

Charlie: This unisex name has English, French, and Germanic origins. It comes from the Old English *ceorl* that means 'man'. In French and German meanings, it stands for 'free man'.

Corey: This unisex name has been borrowed from the Irish. It has several origins. It originated from a Gaelic surname *coire* that means a 'hollow, a seething pool, or a cauldron' and is said to be a dweller near or in a hollow. In German and English, the name means 'God's peace'. It also holds origins with the Norse name of *Kori*.

Dakota: This unisex name is of Native American origin and means 'ally or friend' in the Santee and Yankton-Yanktonai dialects of the Lakota Sioux tribe from the northern Mississippi valley.

Daryl: This unisex name has origins in Old French and Middle English. In French, it is a place name that means 'open'. In English, it means 'dearly loved, and darling'. This name dates back to the 1200s as both a given and surname in France.

Eli: This unisex name is of Hebrew origin and means 'high, elevated, or my God'. Eli was a judge and priest in the Old Testament that raised Samuel who became a prophet. Within the Greek origin, it means 'defender of man'.

Frankie: This unisex name has many different origins. In German, it means 'javelin'. In Latin, it means 'free'. In English, it means 'honest'. Frankie is mostly used as a nickname for Frances, Francine, Francesco, or Frank.

Gray: This unisex name is of English origin. It was used as a nickname for anyone that had gray beards or hair. In Ireland and Scotland, it has been translated from different Gaelic surnames that were derived from *riabhach* meaning 'gray or brindled'.

Harper: This unisex name is of Scottish origin. It originated in the Dalriadan region of Scotland and is part of the Buchanan Clan. Harper was Anglicization of the German name *Harpfer*, meaning to 'play the harp'.

Hayden: This unisex name has many origins. It was an English surname that was derived from different place names. It is derived from the elements *heg* meaning 'hay and *denu* 'valley'; *heg* meaning 'hay' and *dun* meaning 'hill'; *hege* meaning 'hedge' and *dun* meaning 'hill'. It also has Welsh origins from the Hayden meaning 'fire' that was derived from the Celtic name *Aidan*.

Jamie: This unisex name has many origins. It has roots in Hebrew, Scottish, and English. They all mean 'supplanter or seized by the heel'. It is the feminine form or James. There are many different spellings of this name: Jamie, Jaime, and Jamey.

Jesse: This unisex name is of Hebrew origin from the name *Yishai, which* means 'gift'. Jesse is from the Old Testament. He was the father of David. The stem of Jesse is used to describe David's family. Jesse was a wealthy man who held a high position in Bethlehem. Different spellings of this name are Jessie, Jessee or shortened to Jess.

Kennedy: This unisex name is of Gaelic origin and means 'helmeted leader or armored head'. The name is derived from two elements *ceann* meaning 'head' and *eidigh* meaning 'ugly' or *ceann* meaning 'head' and *eide* meaning 'armor' so the name could mean 'helmet headed'.

Morgan: This unisex name comes from Scotland, Brittany, and Wales. The male version *Morcant* is derived from *mor* meaning 'sea' and *cant* meaning 'circle' that means 'sea chief or sea defender'.

Peyton: This unisex name is of English origin and was a place name, meaning 'Paega's town'. It was originally a surname in Sussex. It is a version of Payton.

River: This unisex name is of English origin and means 'river or large creek'. It also has Shakespearean origins. Lord Rivers is Lady Grey's brother in King Henry the Sixth III, and Earl Rivers is King Edward's Queen's brother in King Richard III.

Rudy: This unisex name is of German origin. It is short for Rudolf or Rudiger. Rudiger comes from the Old German *Hruodiger* meaning 'spear fame' or 'fame with a spear'. The name derives from the elements *hroud* meaning 'fame' and *ger* meaning 'spear'. Rudolf means 'famed wolf'.

Stevie: This unisex name is of Greek origin and means 'victorious or crown'. It has been used as a shortened form of Stephanie or Stephen.

Tanner: This unisex name is of English origin. It was a surname that referred to an occupational name. The Old English word *tannere* signified a person who was a tanner of animal skins. They produced leather for everyday items like armor, saddles, horse harnesses, or shoes in medieval times and even before. This word was influenced by the Celtic word for oak tree. The tree bark was used in tanning. The surname was first spelled Tannur in the 1300s.

Taylor: This unisex name is of English origin. It is a surname and comes from the word *tailor*. It ultimately came from the Latin word *taliare* meaning 'to cut'.

Tyler: This unisex name is from English origin and means 'maker of tiles or bricks'. This surname was derived from the old French *tieuleor, tieulier* meaning 'tile maker or tiler' and the Middle English *tyler, tylere* meaning 'a tile or a brick'. The name was originally an occupational name for a brick or tile layer or maker.

West: This unisex name has both German and English origins. From the Middle English, Middle High German west, so it was a topographic name for a person that lived toward the west of a settlement. A regional name for people who migrated from the west.

Winter: This unisex name is of English origins and began as a surname that dates as far back as the ninth century. In Greek mythology, the seasons were placed to give Persephone's time between her lovers on Hades and Earth. Persephone was told to stay with Hades in the Winter until Spring. This name means the 'coldest season of the year'. The Native American meaning is 'bringing of renewal'.

Celtic

Boys

Angus: This boy name is an Anglicized form of the Gaelic *Aonghas*. This is derived from the elements of *one and choice*. A Scottish version is *Aonghus*. *Aonghus* means 'one strength'. This is derived from the elements *one* and *gus* meaning 'energy, strength, or force'. He was the Irish god of youth and love. The Irish form is *Aengus*.

Bowden: This boy name is of Angle-Saxon origin and is from two sources. It can be a place name meaning a 'dweller at the top of a hill' or from the Old English phrase, *befan dune* that means 'above the hill'. It could also be from any place called Bowdon or Bowden. There are places in Scotland from the Gaelic both *an duin* that translates to 'house on the hill'.

Driscoll: This boy name is of Irish origin. It is a reduced for of the Gaelic *O' hEidirsceoil* meaning 'descendant of the messenger', from *eidirsceol* meaning 'news bearer, intermediary, and go between'.

Fergus: This boy name is of Irish origin and means 'man of vigor'. It is derived from the elements *fear* meaning 'man' and *gus* meaning 'vigor'. This is a popular Irish or Scottish given name. It originally came from the Proto-Celtic elements *wiros* meaning 'man' and *gustus* meaning 'choice, force, or vigor'. The first reference is to a Pictish king. The surname of Fergusson or Ferguson is normal across Scotland but more in Ayrshire and Perthshire. In Ireland, the Ferris family gets its surname from *O'Fearghusa*.

Kegan: This boy name is of Irish, Gaelic, and Celtic origin. They all mean 'fiery and small'.

Maddox: This boy name is of Welsh origin. It originally was a surname meaning son of Madoc. Madoc or Madog was a Welsh prince that supposedly sailed to the New World three hundred years before Columbus did. The name means 'fortunate' and is derived from the element *mad*.

Owyn: This boy name is of Irish, Welsh, and Celtic origins and means 'young fighter'. It is a variation of Owen.

Sloane: This boy name is of Irish origin. It was used as a surname but was Anglicized from the Irish *O'Sluaghain*. *Sluaghhadain* is a version of the ancient Gaelic name *Sluaghadh* that means 'raid'. Therefore, Sloane means 'little raider'.

Tiernay: This boy name is of Irish origin. It means 'chief or lord' and implies 'lord of the household'. It is the Anglicized form of the surname *Tighearnach*.

Weylin: This boy name is of Celtic origin and means 'son of the wolf'. It is a variation of Waylon.

Girls

Brygid: This girl name is of Gaelic origin and means 'strength or exalted one'. It is a variation of the name, Bridget.

Cordelia: This girl name is of Celtic origin. It became famous as the heroine in Shakespeare's King Lear. The character was based on queen Cordelia. The meaning is uncertain but could be derived from the Latin *cor* meaning 'heart'. It is also linked with the Welsh name *Creiddylad* meaning 'jewel of the sea'. It could also come from the French *Coeur de lion* meaning 'heart of a lion'.

Etain: This girl name is of Irish origin and means 'jealousy'. The Irish myth holds Etain as a beautiful fairy who was turned into a scarlet fly by a jealous queen. She was blown off an ocean for several years. When she was able to come back to Ireland, she fell into some wine and was swallowed by a woman who wanted a child. Etain was reborn and married a King of Ireland.

Fiona: This girl name is of Gaelic origin and means 'fair or white'. Fiona is the most well-known in a group of Gaelic names. This is ironic since it is without genuine roots. It was first found in the *Ossianic* poem of James Macpherson. It became popular in the late 1800s as a feminine pen name for a Scottish writer.

Gwyndolin: This girl name is of Welsh origin and means 'white ring'. It is derived from the elements *gwen* meaning 'blessed, white, fair' and *dolen* meaning 'ring'. This is a mythical queen who fought her husband in battle and defeated him.

Kaedence: This girl name is of Celtic origin and means 'to march in rhythm'.

Lyonesse: This girl name is of Celtic origin and means 'little lion'.

Morrigan: This girl name is of Irish origin. It is derived from *Mor Rioghain* that means 'great queen'. In an Irish myth, she is a goddess of war and took the form of a cow.

Oriana: This girl name is of Latin origin meaning 'rising sun'. This medieval name is exotic and strong. She was the love of knight Amadis.

Venetia: This girl name is of Celtic origin. It is a place name the means 'blessed'. It is a form of Gwyneth.

Unisex

Arleigh: This unisex name is of Old English origin. It is a variant of Arley and Harley. It made its way into popularity with the Scots and became one of the top Celtic names. It means 'vow or pledge'.

Arlyss: This unisex name is of Welsh origin meaning 'snowdrop'. It is a variation of Eirlys. This name is attractive and has a lot of flair and character.

Bevan: This unisex name is of Welsh, Gaelic, and Celtic origin. It is derived from *ab-evan* that means 'son of Evan'. The Gaelic meaning is 'fair lady'. The Celtic origin is 'youthful warrior'.

Brennan: This unisex name is of Gaelic and Irish origin. It comes from the surname Brennan which in Irish is spelled *o'Braonain* and means the 'descendant of Braonan'. The Gaelic personal name *Braonan* comes from the Irish *braon* that means 'sorrow'. In other cases, the name may have come from the name, Brendan.

Caradoc: This unisex name is of Welsh origin and means 'amiable, affection'. In Celtic origin, it means 'dearly loved'. This ancient Celtic name is shared with a Knight of the Round Table and a Welsh King. This name was very common in the Middle Ages. This name appears in Welsh Triads as Arthur's chief elder and one of the knights of the Britain Island.

Carrington: This unisex name is of Celtic origin and is a surname and place name. It means 'town of the marsh'.

Kerwin: This unisex name is of Irish, Gaelic, and Celtic origin. It means 'small black one' in Irish, 'little black one' in Gaelic, and 'dark skinned' in Celtic.

Makenna: This unisex name is of Gaelic origin. It was originally a surname *Mac Cionaodha* that means 'son of Cionaodh'. It is a variation of McKenna and means 'happy one'.

Sheridan: This unisex name is an Irish surname that is derived from *O' Sirideain* that means 'descendant of *Siridean*'. The elements *O* meaning 'descendant of' and *Sirideain* is a nickname for 'elf'. It is possible since elves were known to be mischievous creatures, someone was given this nickname because they were somewhat mischievous as well. In Gaelic, the name *Siridean* means 'searcher'.

Tiernan: This unisex name is of Irish origin and means 'little lord'. It comes from an Old Gaelic name *MacTighearnain* that means 'son of Tierna'. This name means 'master or lord'. Variations of this surname are O'Tiernan, MacTiernan, McTiernan, and Tiernan.

Nordic

Boys

Bard: This boy name is of Norwegian origin. It is from the Old Norse *Bardr* that comes from the elements *badu,* meaning 'battle' and *fridr,* meaning 'peace'. Therefore, it means 'battle against peace'.

Calder: This boy name is of Old Norse origin via Scotland. It is a place name from any places like Cawdor, Caldor, or Calder. Calder in Thurso was recorded in the early 1200s with the spelling *Kalfadal* which is derived from the elements *kalfr* meaning 'calf' and *dalr* meaning 'valley'. From the Welsh origin, it is derived from the elements *caled* meaning 'hard or violent' and *dwfr* meaning 'stream or water'. So, its meaning could be 'valley of the calf' or 'violent water'.

Eirik: This boy name is of Norse origin and means 'eternal ruler' or 'forever strong'. This is a variation of Eric. It was once popular with Scandinavian royalty since many kings of Denmark, Norway, and Sweden used it.

Gandalf: This boy name is from Norse Mythology origin and means elf with a wand. It comes from the elements gandr, meaning cane, staff, or wand

and alfr, meaning elf. The famous bearer of the name is the beloved character in the novel, *The Lord of the Rings* written by J.R.R. Tolkien.

Ivar: This boy name is of Danish, Norwegian, and Swedish origins. It is an Old Norse name *Ivarr*. It is derived from elements *yr* meaning 'bow or yew' and *arr* meaning 'warrior'. Therefore, it means 'warrior with a bow'. It was brought to England by the Scandinavian invaders during the Middle Ages. It was adopted by Wales, Scotland, and Ireland.

Kensley: This boy name has origins in both Old Norse and Gaelic meaning from a 'clearing with a spring'. It is derived from the elements *kelda* that means 'well or spring' and the Old English word meaning *leah* that means 'wood or clearing'. It is a place name showing the bearer comes from near a clearing with a spring.

Odin: This boy name is of Old Norse origin and means 'fury'. It is derived from the element *odr* that means 'inspiration or fury'. *Odin* was the god of death, wisdom, and war in Norse mythology.

Stig: This boy name has origins in Old Norse and Danish. It is a variation of *Stigr* and originates from the Old Norse meaning 'route'.

Sven: This boy name is of Old Norse origin and means boy. Sven is from Scandinavia of Old Norse origins. It derives from the element *sven* that means 'boy'.

Viggo: This boy name is of Old Norse origin and means battle. It is derived from the element *vig* meaning 'war or fight'.

Girls

Aslog: This girl name is from Old Norse and Danish origins and means 'woman engaged to God'. It is a variation of the name *Aslaug*. It derives from the element *ass* meaning 'God' and *laug* meaning 'betrothed woman'.

Astrid: This girl name is of Old Norse origin and means 'divine beauty'. It is derived from the elements *ass* meaning 'God' and *fridr* meaning 'beloved or beautiful'. It's more popular with Scandinavian languages because of the creator of Pippi Longstocking's author Astrid Lindgren.

Brenna: This girl name is of Old Norse origin and means 'sword'. It is a variation of Brenda. It is the feminine of the Old Norse Brandr that means 'sword that was brought to Britain' during the Middle Ages.

Freja: This girl name is of Swedish, Old Norse, and Danish origins. It means 'like a lady'. It is very popular in Scandinavia but rare elsewhere. It is derived from the element *Freyja* meaning 'lady'. This name belongs to the goddess of death, war, beauty, and love in Norse mythology. She said most of the heroes that were slain were brought to her realm in Folkvangr. With her father Njord and brother Freyr. Some connect her to the goddess Frigg. In Denmark and Sweden, it is spelled Freja. In Norway, it is spelled Froja.

Ingrid: This girl name is of Old Norse origin and means 'beautiful goddess'. Ing was another name for Freyr in Norse mythology. She was an important god of fertility, weather, and farming. Ingrid is an extremely popular name in the Scandinavian countries

Ragna: This girl name is of Swedish, Old Norse, and Danish origins and means 'giving advice'. This is a shortened form of Old Norse names that began with element 'regin' meaning 'counsel or advice'.

Sigfrid: This girl name is of Old Norse and Norwegian origins and means 'marvelous victory'. It is a variation of Sigrid. It is derived from the elements *sigr* meaning 'victory' and *fridr* meaning 'fair or beautiful'.

Thora: This girl name is of Old Norse origin and means 'like thunder'. It is the feminine form or Thor who is the Norse god of thunder, power, and war. Thora was a wife of Ragnar Lodbrok who was a king of Denmark in Norse mythology.

Tyra: This girl name is of Old Norse origin and means 'like thunder'. It is the feminine form of Tyr who is the Norse god of justice and war.

Unisex

Beau: This unisex name is of French origin and means 'beautiful person'. It was used as a form of endearment for a girl or a nickname for a good man.

Dagny: This unisex name is of Old Norse origin and means 'new day started'. It is derived from the elements *dagr* meaning 'day' and *ny* meaning 'new'.

Haley: This unisex name is of English origin and means 'meadow of hay'. It is a variant of Haley. It is derived from Old English surname. It comes from *heg* meaning 'hay' and *leah* meaning 'clearing'. It could mean 'heroine' in the Old Norse language.

Karina: This unisex name is of Swedish, Russian, Polish, Norwegian, Greek, and Danish origins. It means pure or chaste. It is one of the most popular names with many different spellings over the entire world. It could be a variation of Katherine.

Loki: This unisex name is of Old Norse origin and means 'trickster'. Loki is the name of the trickster god in Norse mythology. He used fire and magic against people. He became very evil, and the other gods chained him to a rock. It is used as a nickname for someone who is thought to be a cheater.

Mikko: This unisex name is of Hebrew and Finnish origins and means 'which man is like God'? It is a variant of Michael. Can be spelled, Mika.

Montana: This unisex name is of Latin origin and means from 'a hilly land'. It is derived from a Spanish word that means 'mountain'. It is also used as a surname.

Rayne: This unisex name is of English origin and means 'woman of rain'. Could be based on the French word *reine* that means 'queen'.

Signy: This unisex name is of Danish, Norwegian, and Swedish origins and means 'latest victory'. It is derived from elements *sigr* meaning 'victory' and *ny* meaning 'new'. In Norse legends, it was the wife of Siggeir and the sister of Sigmund.

Ziv: This unisex name is of Hebrew origin and means 'shining'. It is the ancient name of a month in the Jewish calendar.

German

Boys

Anton: This boy name is of German origin. It is from the Roman name *Antonius*. The most memorable person within the Roman family was Marcus Antonius who ruled the Roman Empire with Augustus. When their friendship went south, his mistress Cleopatra and he were attacked, and they forced them to commit suicide, as stated in Shakespeare's tragedy, *Antony and Cleopatra*.

Barney: This boy name is of German origin. It is a shortened version of Bernard. It is derived from the element *bern* meaning 'bear' and *hard* meaning 'hardy or brave'. The Normans were the one who brought it to England, and it replaced the Old English name Beornheard. Several saints bore the name Bernard. Saint Bernard of Menthon built hospices in the 900s in the Swiss Alps. Saint Bernard of Clairvaux was a doctor of the church and a theologian in the 1300s.

Conrad: This boy name is of German origin. It is derived from the elements *kuoni* meaning 'brave' and *rad* meaning 'counsel'. A bishop and saint who lived in the 900s in Konstanz that is located in southern Germany. Several medieval Kings and

Dukes bore this name as well. It was used some time during the Middle Ages in England but has become more common in the 1800s when Germany reintroduced the name.

Dirk: This boy name is of German origin. It is from the German name Theodoric meaning 'ruler of the people'. It is derived from the elements *theud* meaning 'people' and *ric* meaning 'ruler or power'. Theodoric the Great who was a king in the 500s of Ostrogoth and became ruler of Italy. His name became Romanized and was recorded as Theodoricus. The Gothic spelling is Diudreiks.

Ferdinand: This boy name is of German origin. It comes from Ferdinando which is the Old Spanish form of the Germanic name with the elements *fardi* meaning 'journey' and *nand* meaning 'brave or daring'. The Visigoths brought it to the Iberian Peninsula where royal families of Portugal and Spain began using it. It was popular with the Roman Empire, the Habsburg royal family, and Austria.

Hans: This boy name is of Scandinavian, Dutch, and German origins. It is a shortened version of Johannes. Johannes is from the Latin Ioannes meaning John. John is from the Hebrew name Yochanan meaning 'Yahweh is gracious'.

Jansen: This boy name is of Flemish, Low German, and Dutch origins. It was a surname meaning 'son of Jan'. It is derived from the name Johannes.

Kiefer: This boy name is of German origin. It is an occupational name for an overseer of wine cellars from the elements *kuofe* meaning 'barrel or vat'. It is also a version of the Middle High German *kiffen* 'to quarrel' and became a nickname for a person who likes to bicker. It is from the German *kiefer* meaning 'pine tree'. It is derived from two elements *kein* and *forhe* both meaning 'pine tree'.

Leo: This boy name is of German origin. It is derived from the Latin *leo* meaning 'lion' which is a version of Leon. It became popular with Christians as it was the name of 13 popes.

Pepin: This boy name is of German origin. It was originally a surname in northwest Germany around the city of Cologne. It is derived from the word *pepin* or *pipin* meaning 'seed of a fruit' and is an occupational name for a 'grower of fruit trees or gardener'.

Girls

Adalie: This girl name is of German origin. It means 'noble one' or 'God is my refuge'. It is a variation of Adalia which is Old German and Hebrew. It is also a variation of Adela which is Old German.

Bernadette: This girl name is of German origin. It is a feminine version of the name Bernard. It comes from the Germanic element *bern* meaning 'bear' combined with *hard* meaning 'hardy or brave'. The Normans introduced it to England, and it replaced *Beornheard*.

Delmira: This girl name is of German origin. It means 'famous or noble'. It is a variation of Delma and has the nickname of Adelma.

Farica: This girl name is of German origin and means 'peaceful ruler'. It is a shortened version of Frederica. It is made up of the elements *frid* meaning 'peace' and *ric* meaning 'power or ruler'. This name is common in German speaking regions.

Geneva: This girl name is of German origin. It comes from the medieval name *Genovefa*. It is derived from the elements *kuni* meaning 'family' or 'kin' and *wefa* meaning 'woman or wife'. Another origin is Gaulish from the Celtic element *genos* meaning 'family or kin'.

Georgia: This girls name is a variation of the German name, Georgina, which is the feminine version of the name, George. The word was derived from the Greek word *georgos*, which means 'farmer or earthworker'. The name became popular in England when the German-born George I took the British throne.

Jenell: The name Jenell is a German name which means 'kindness, knowledge, and understanding'. In Latin and English, the name means 'maiden' and is a variation of the name, Janelle.

Joli: This name comes from French origins. While in France it is not often given as a given name. The name means 'beautiful' in French and 'pretty and cheerful' in English.

Katrina: The name Katrina is a variation of Katherine. It is derived from the Greek name *Aikaterine*. It is debated as to where this name originally came from. It could be the Greek name *Hekaterine*, which was taken from *hekateros*, which means 'each of the two'. And it's also believed to have come from the Goddess Hecate.

Lorelei: This name comes from a Germanic name that means 'luring rock'. The name is derived from a rocky headland that is located on the Rhine River.

Unisex

Ade: The name Ade is a variation of the German name, Adalwold, which means 'noble wolf'. Broken down, it comes from the element *adal* meaning 'noble' and wulf meaning 'wolf'. It was a popular name among Swedish Kings.

Al: This name mainly started out as a nickname for somebody named Albert, but has since become a popular choice for a given name. It comes from the German name Adalbert, which is made up of the element *adal*, meaning 'noble' and 'beraht' meaning *bright*. This was a common medieval German royalty name.

Bernie: The name Bernie comes from the name Bernard. The name was derived from the Germanic element *bern* meaning 'bear' and mixed with *hard* meaning 'brave and hardy'.

Claiborne: Not much is known about this name. It has origins in both Germany and England. In German, it means 'boundary with clover'. It's a common English surname that was found in the Norfolk and southeast area of England, possibly meaning 'clay by a river'.

Clovis: This name is a shortened version of the name *Clodovicus*, which is the Latinized form of the German name *Chlodevech*, which is also changed to Ludwig. It comes from the elements *hlud* meaning 'famous' and *wig* which means 'battle or war'.

Fritzi: This name comes from a diminutive form of the German name, Friederike, which comes from the name, Frederick. The name means 'peaceful ruler'. It comes from the elements *frid* meaning 'peace' and *ric* meaning 'power or ruler'.

Halle: The name Halle came about from the German surname, Halle, which is a 'cognate of Hall'. This name was derived from an Old English word, heal, which means 'hall or manor'. This name was given to a person that worked or lived in a manor.

Karlyn: This name has both English and Old German origins. Karlyn means 'free man' and is a variation of the Old German name, Carlene and the English name, Karleen.

Malin: This name a shorter variation of the name Magdalene. The name originated from a title that meant 'of Magdala'. The New Testament character Mary Magdalene was named such because she was from Magdala, which is a village on the Sea of Galilee.

Rory: The name Rory has become gained popularity as a German name over the past few centuries. The names origin is Gaelic. It comes from the Irish name, Ruairi, and the Scottish name, Ruairidah. The name means 'red king'.

Historical

Boys

Amadeus: The name Amadeus means 'love of God'. The name was derived from the Latin word *amare* which means 'to love' and *Deus* which means 'God'. The famous composer, Wolfgang Amadeus Mozart, carried this name.

Aurelius: This name is a common name from early saints. It started as a Roman family name and was derived from the Latin word *aureus* which means 'gilded or golden'.

Cassius: This name started out as a Roman family name that was probably derived from the Latin word *cassus* which means 'vain or empty'. This was also a common name given to saints.

Demetrius: This name is a Latin version of the Greek name, Demetrios, which came from the name of the Greek Goddess, Demeter. Many early saints were given this name, and Seleucid kingdom and the Kings of Macedon used this name.

Felix: This name is derived from a famous Roman cognomen, which means 'successful or lucky' in Latin. It was given as an agnomen to the 1st-century Roman general Sulla. In the New Testament, it belongs to the governor of Judea. This was a popular name for early Christians because of its meaning.

Magnus: This name is derived from a late Latin word that means 'great'. A 7th-century saint bore this name. It gained popularity in Scandinavia with the 11th century Norwegian King Magnus I.

Septimus: This name is a Roman given name, which in Latin it means 'seventh'. This name was given to the Emperor Septimus Severus, which was a patron of arts and letters.

Severus: This name is derived from a Roman family name, and in Latin it means 'stern'. This was a popular name among early saints.

Thor: This name comes from an Old Norse word which means 'thunder', which came from an early Germanic word. Thor is the god of thunder, storms, strength, and war in Norse mythology, and is the son of Odin.

Urban: The name Urban comes from the Latin name *Urbanus* which means 'city dweller'. Paul mentions this name in one of his New Testament epistles. It has been a name of eight popes.

Girls

Aeliana: The name Aeliana is the female form of the name, Aelianus. Aelianus is a Roman cognomen which they derived from the name, Aelius. This family name was possibly taken from the Greek word *helios* which means 'the sun'.

Atarah: This name in Hebrew means crown. Atarah was the wife of Jerahmeel in the Old Testament.

Crispina: This name is the feminine form of the name Crispin. This was a Roman cognomen, Crispinus, which they got from the name, Crispus. A 3rd century Roman, Saint Crispin, was martyred along with his twin broth in Gaul. They are considered to be the patron saints of shoemakers.

Delicia: This name was either derived from the Latin word *deliciae* which means 'pleasure or delight' or the English word delicious. This name is a rarely used name and has only been popular since the early 20th century.

Felicia: The name Felicia is the female version of the Latin name, Felicius, which is derived from the name, Felix. It has occasionally been used in England since the Middle Ages.

Jonet: The name Jonet is an obsolete Scottish spelling of the name, Janet. Janet is a medieval version of the name, Jane, which is a feminine version of the name, John. The meaning of the name goes back to the Hebrew name, Yochanan, which means 'Yahweh is gracious'.

Lucilla: This name is the Latin diminutive of Lucia. A 3rd-century saint that was martyred in Rome had this name. The name is derived from the Latin word *lux* which means 'light'.

Minerva: This name is possibly derived from the Latin word *mens* which means 'intellect', but is more likely to have an Etruscan origin. In Roman mythology, Minerva was the goddess of war and wisdom, which is basically the equivalent of the Greek Goddess, Athena. It has been a popular name since after the English Renaissance.

Sabina: This name is the female version of Sabinus, which is a Roman cognomen that means 'Sabine' in Latin. Ancient people that lived in central Italy were known as the Sabines and their lands were taken by the Romans after many wars.

Viviana: The name, Viviana, is the female version of Vivianus. The 4th-century saint, Saint Viviana, was a martyr. The name was derived from the Latin word *vivus* which means 'alive'.

Unisex

Alva: This unisex name is derived from the name, Alf. It comes from the Old Norse word *alfr* meaning 'elf'. The name could also be a variation of the name, Alvah, which in Hebrew means 'his highness'.

Angel: This name is derived from the Latin medieval masculine name, Angelus, which came from the name that was given to heavenly creature. That name came from the Greek word *angelos* which means 'messenger'. In the English-speaking world, it's not that popular.

Brook: The name, Brook, started as an English surname. The surname was given to people that lived near a brook, making the meaning of the name 'the one who lives near a brook' or 'a running stream'.

Cheyenne: This name comes from the Dakota word, shahiyena, which means 'red speakers'. This name comes from Native Americans who are from the Great Plains. The Dakotas gave the Cheyenne this name because their language was unrelated to theirs.

Dee: The name, Dee, in Welsh is often a nickname for a person considered swarthy, and comes from the Welsh word *du* meaning 'black or dark'. In

Irish, it is a variation of Daw. In Scotland and England, it is a habitational name of a person that lived near the banks on the Dee River in Cheshire or in Scotland. Both of these were derived from a Celtic word that means goddess or sacred.

Dusty: This name was often given to people as a nickname if they seemed to be dusty. It is also a variation of Dustin. This name is derived from an English surname which came from the Old Norse name, Torsten, which means Thor's stone.

Gale: This name is a shortened version of the name Abigail, which comes from the Hebrew name 'Avigayil, which means 'my father is joy'. It also comes from an English surname that was taken from a Middle English word, gaile, which means 'jovial'.

Jackie: This name most often comes from the names Jacqueline or Jack. Jack is the medieval diminutive of John, which comes from the Hebrew name, Yochana, which means 'Yahweh is gracious'. Jacqueline is the feminine version of Jacques, which is the French form of the name, Jacob. The name means 'may God protect.

Johnnie: This name is a diminutive of the name, John. The name, John, comes the Latin word Johannes, which comes from the Greek name,

Joannes, which comes from the Hebrew name *Yochanan*, which means 'Yahweh is gracious'.

Lee: The name Lee started out as a surname that was derived from an Old English word leah, which means 'clearing'. Lee means 'dweller by the wood or clearing'. Lee is commonly used in combination names like Lee-Ann and Bobby-Lee.

Most Common

Boys

Alexander: This name is the Latinized form of the Greek name, Alexandros. This name means 'defending men', which comes from the Greek word *alexo* meaning 'to defend, help' and *aner* meaning 'man'. This was also another name for the hero Paris in Greek mythology.

Benjamin: The name Benjamin comes from the Hebrew name *Binyamin*. It means 'son of the right hand' or 'son of the south'. In the Old Testament, the youngest son of Jacob was Benjamin and a founder of a southern Hebrew tribe.

Carter: The name Carter started out being used for the surname of a cart driver. It is of English descent and it means 'Driver of a cart'.

Cole: The origin of this name is Anglo-Saxon. This name came from a surname that in Old English was the byname Cola. This name means charcoal and used to be given to people that had dark features.

Daniel: The name Daniel originates from the old Hebrew name *Daniyyel,* which means 'God is my judge'. In the Old Testament, Daniel is a Hebrew prophet. The name became popular during the Middle Ages in England due to the biblical character.

Dylan: This name comes from Wales, and it's derived from the element *dy,* which means 'great' and *llanw* which means 'tide and flow'. Dylan, in Welsh mythology, was a hero or god that was associated with the sea.

Greyson: This name is a variation of the English name Grayson. It comes from an English surname that meant 'son of the steward'. This name was derived from the Middle English word, *greyve,* which means 'steward'.

Jackson: The name Jackson started out as an English surname that means 'son of Jack'. In English, Jack is the diminutive form of John.

Jacob: This name originated from the Latin word *Iacobus* which was derived from the Greek word *Iakobos,* which was derived from the Hebrew name *Ya'aqov.* Jacob in the Old Testament is the son of Rebecca and Isaac. During the Middle Ages in England, Jacob was viewed as a mainly Jewish name. It started being used as a Christian name after the Protestant Reformation.

Juan: This name is the Manx and Spanish version of the name Johannes, which is the name, John.

The name John dates back to the Hebrew name *Yochanan*, which means 'Yahweh is gracious'.

Matthew: This name is an English form of the word Matthaios, which is a Greek form of a Hebrew name, *Mattityahu,* which means 'gift of Yahweh'. In the Bible Matthew is one of the 12 apostles.

Miles: This name comes from the Germanic name, Milo. The name was introduced to England by the Normans in the form of the name, Miles. The actual definition of the name is not certain. It may be connected with the Slavic element *milu* which means 'gracious'. It could also date back to the Latin word miles, meaning soldier.

Oliver: This name is derived from the Norman French name Olivier, which was a form of a Germanic name Alfher, or the Norse name, Olaf. The spelling of the name was changed over time because of its association with the Latin word *olive* which means 'olive tree'.

Roman: The name Roman comes from a late Latin name *Romanus*, which means 'Roman'. The name Roman means to be of Rome.

Samuel: Samuel comes from the Hebrew name *Shemu'el* which may mean "God has heard' or 'name of God'. Samuel, in the Old Testament, was the last ruling judge. Samuel becomes a popular Christian name after the Protestant Reformation.

Theodore: This name originated from the Greek name Theodoros, which means 'gift of God.' It is broken down into the Greek words *theos* meaning God and *doron* meaning gift.

Tristan: This name comes from the French form of the Pictish name, Drustan, which is also a diminutive form of Drust. The name's spelling has been changed because of the Latin *tristis* which means sad.

Vincent: The name Vincent comes from the Roman name, Vincentius, which comes from the Latin *vincere* which means 'to conquer'. This was a very popular name for the early Christians, and many saints bore this name.

Wesley: This English name comes from an old surname that was derived from a place name that, in Old English, means 'west meadow'. At one time, the name was given in honor of the Methodist faith founder, John Wesley.

Weston: This name is of English origin. It started out as a surname that was given to people who lived west of the town. It comes from an Old English word.

Girls

Aurora: The name Aurora comes from a Latin word that means dawn. In Roman mythology, Aurora was the Goddess of the morning. It has been used as a name since the Renaissance

Chloe: The name Chloe means 'green shoot' in Greek, which refers to the new plants that grow in spring. The Greek Goddess Demeter used this as an epithet. The name is also mentioned in the New Testament in one of Paul's epistles.

Daisy: This is an English name that was taken from the pretty white flower. It was originally derived from the Old English word *dœgeseage* which means 'day eye'. The word first appeared as a given name during the 1800s, which was also at the same time as many other flowers and plants were given names.

Elizabeth: This name was derived from the Greek name, Elisabet, which was derived from the Hebrew name *Elisheva* which means 'my God is abundance' or 'my God is an oath'. In the Old Testament, the Hebrew version of the name appears where Elisheba is the wife of Aaron. The Greek form makes an appearance in the New Testament where John the Baptist's mother is Elizabeth.

Evelyn: The name Evelyn comes from an English surname, which came from Aveline; a given name. When the name was first used as a given name in the 17th century, it was used more often for boys.

Grace: This name comes from the English word grace, which was originated from the Latin word *gratia*. The Puritans created this name in the 17th century as one of their virtue names.

Harmony: This is an English name that was derived from the English word harmony. The word was originally derived from the Greek word *harmonia*. Within Greek mythology, Harmonia is the Goddess of harmony, happy marriages, sisterhood, and brotherhood. Her parents are Ares, god of war, and Aphrodite, goddess of love. Harmony is a musical term that signifies a note combination that is played at the same time that gives a pretty melody.

Hannah: This name originates with the Hebrew name, Channah, which means 'grace or favor'. In the Old Testament, Elkanah's wife had this name. Hannah didn't become a common name until after the Protestant Reformation.

Katherine: This name comes from the Greek name Aikaterine. It is debated as to where it originated and is believed could have come from an early Greek name *hekaterine*, which means each of the two, or from the Goddess, Hecate. It may also be from the Greek word *aikia*, which means torture, or it may also be from the Coptic name that means 'my consecration of your name.' Early Christians associated the name with the Greek word *katharos*, which means pure.

Kimberly: The name Kimberly comes from a city in South Africa, named, Kimberley. This city was named after Lord Kimberley. The name is a variation of Cyneburg, which means royal fortress. Broken down, it comes from the Old English cyne, which means royal, and burg, meaning fortress.

Layla: This name comes from an Arabic word meaning night. The 7th-century poems, Layla was the romantic interest of a poet known as Qays. This became a popular romance within medieval Persia and Arabia.

Lily: This name is derived from the Latin word *lilium*. The name comes from the flower, which is a symbol of purity.

Madison: This name started out as an English surname, which means 'son of Maud'. The name became a popular name for girls when the 1984 movie "Splash" came out.

Maria: This name is the Latin form of the Greek name *Mapiaz*, which comes from the Hebrew name Mary. Maria is the most common form of the name Mary in most European languages and the secondary form in many other languages like English. In some countries, Maria is used as a masculine middle name. The meaning is not completely known, but it could mean 'wished for child,' 'sea of bitterness,' or 'rebelliousness.' But it is most likely taken from an Egyptian name, broken down to *mry*, meaning beloved, or *mr*, meaning love.

Melanie: This name comes from Mélanie, which is the French version of the Latin Melania, which they derived from the Greek word melaina, which means dark or black. A 5th-century Roman saint was given this name; she gave all of her money to charity. It became a popular name during the Middle Ages in France.

Rachel: The name Rachel is derived from the Hebrew name Rachel, which means ewe. This is the favorite wife of Jacob in the Old Testament, and she is the mother of Benjamin, and Joseph. She was also Jacob's first wife, Leah's, little sister. This was a common name for Jews during the Middle Ages, but it didn't become a Christian name until after the Protestant Reformation.

Rose: This name started out as a Norman form of a German name, which was made up of *hruod*, which means 'fame', and *heid*, which means 'type, kind, and sort'. The English was introduced to this name by the Normans in the forms of Rohese and Roese. From early on it has been associated with the good smelling flower rose, which came from the Latin word *rosa*. When the name became popular again in the 19th century, it was probably due to the flower.

Scarlett: This name came from the surname that they used for a person that made or sold clothes that had been made from scarlet, which is a type of cloth. This name was derived from the Persian word *saghrilat*.

Valerie: This name is the German and English version of Valeria and Czech version of Valérie. The name Valeria is the female form of Valerius, which comes from the Latin word *valere*, which means 'to be strong'. Many early saints bore this name.

Victoria: In Latin, this name means victory, and is borne of the Roman Goddess of victory. This name is the female version of the name, Victorius. The first use of this name was from a North African martyr and saint of the 4th century.

Unisex

Alex: This name is a shortened version of any name that begins with Alex. Lately, it has become popular as a given name for both boys and girls, instead of just used as a nickname. The name means 'to defend or help'.

Drew: The name Drew is derived from the name Andrew, which is the English version of the Greek Andreas, which they derived from *andreios*, which means 'manly and masculine'. Andre was the first disciple of Jesus in the New Testament.

Jaden: The name Jaden is a recently invented name, became popular in the 1990s, and used the popular aden suffix that is found in many other names. It is also, sometimes, considered to be derived from the name Jadon which means 'he will judge' or 'thankful' in Hebrew.

Jordan: This name comes from the name of the river that runs between Israel and Jordan. The name comes from the Hebrew word, Yarden, and it was derived from *yarad* which means 'flow down or descend'. Jesus Christ was baptized in the river by John the Baptist.

Kyle: While this name is seen more for boys, it has recently become popular for both sexes. It originated from the Scottish surname that was derived from the Gaelic word *caol,* which means 'strait, channel, or narrow'.

Parker: This name originated in England as an occupational surname for people. It means 'keeper of the park'.

Nico: The name Nico comes from the name Nicholas or Nicodemus. It's derived from the Greek name *Nikolaos* which means 'victory of the people'. This is broken down into the Greek word *nike* which means 'victory' and *laos* which means 'people'.

Regan: This name is believed to have Celtic origins, but the meaning is unknown. Shakespeare used the name in his play "King Lear" which is found in early British legends. Regan also comes from the name Reagan, which is an Irish surname and an Anglicized form of *Ó Riagain* which means 'descendant of Riagan'.

Sawyer: This name comes from a Middle English surname that was an occupational name meaning 'sawer of wood'. This name is probably most popular in the book *The Adventures of Tom Sawyer* by Mark Twain.

Skyler: The name Skyler is derived from the name *Schuyler*. The change in the spelling happened because of the name Tyler and the word sky. In Dutch, *Schuyler* is a surname that means 'scholar'.

Most Unusual

Boys

Ace: This unique name is typically given to people as a nickname. It originated from an English word that means 'highest rank'. The English word was derived from a Latin word that means 'first-rate or unity'.

Axel: The name Axel is a Medieval Danish form of the name, Absalon. Absalom comes from the Hebrew name, Avshalom, which means 'my father is peace'. Within the Old Testament, Absolom is the son of King David.

Constantine: This name comes from the Latin name *Constantinus*, and is derived from *Constans*. The Roman Emperor Constantine the Great was the first emperor to adopt Christianity. He took the empire to Byzantium and renamed it Constantinople, which has been renamed to Istanbul.

Finn: Finn comes from Irish origin and is an older form of *Fionn*. The name means 'white or fair'. Finn is the most common Anglicized form.

Gunner: This name is derived from the Scandinavian name, Gunther, which means 'bold warrior'. This comes from the Old Norse name

Gunnar which was derived from the word *gunnr* which means 'battle, strife, and war'.

Jett: The name Jett comes from the English word, Jet. This name can refer to the flying aircraft of the same name or a black mineral or color.

Kane: The name Kane is derived from the Irish name, Cathan. Cathan came from the Gaelic word *cath* which means 'battle'. In Hawaii and Japan, the name is transformed into a two-syllable name pronounced, KA-ned. In Welsh, it means 'beautiful', in Japanese, it means 'golden', and in Hawaiian, it means 'man of the Eastern sky.'

Rocco: This name is Germanic, and was derived from the element *hrok* which means 'rest'. This is the same name of a 14th-century French saint that helped nurse plague victims but ended up contracting it as well. He is now considered the patron saint of the sick.

Titus: This name is a Roman given name that comes from unknown meaning, but it could be related to the Latin word *titulus* which means 'title of honor'. A more likely origin is Oscan, since the name come from the legendary Sabine King, Titus Tatius.

Zane: The origin of this name is Semitic, where it is a variation of Jon which means 'God's gracious gift.' Another meaning of the word is 'good' when used in this masculine form.

Girls

Addilyn: This girl name is French in origin and comes from the names, Adeline and Adele, which mean 'kind and noble'. Addilyn can also be a variation of the name Madelyn, which in France came from Madeleine which was in honor of Mary Magdalene.

Aria: The origin of this pretty girl name is Italian where it means 'literally, air, or melody and song'. Aria is a vocal solo which is typically performed during operas. It has only been used as a name since the 20th century.

Bronwyn: This name has both Irish and Welsh origins. The Welsh feminine version is spelled Bronwen, while the Irish feminine version is spelled Bronwyn. Both versions mean 'pure and dark', 'white breasted', and 'white breast'.

Camari: This name comes from Gaelic origins. Originally a surname that meant 'crooked nose', broken down it comes from *cam* which means 'crooked' and *sron* which means 'nose'. This is the same as the name Cameron.

Diem: The origin of Diem is Latin, and means 'day'. In Vietnamese, the name means 'pretty'.

Effie: Effie is of Scottish origin. It comes from the Anglicized form of the word *Oighrig*, which means 'new speckled one'.

Ember: The name Ember comes for the Old English word *œmyrge,* which comes from the proto-Germanic word *aima* meaning 'ashes'. The word Ember means 'glowing coal in a dying fire.' This given name was first recorded in the 1800s, which most likely came as a transfer of the surname, Ember.

Fleur: The origin of Fleur comes from a French word meaning 'flower'. Fleur was introduced to the English through the author, John Galsworthy, who gave it to a character in his books.

Gianna: This unique girl's name is a feminized version of the Latin name, John. The origin of Gianna comes from Italy as a diminutive of Giovanna. It means 'the Lord is gracious'.

Harlyn: Harlyn is the feminized version of the name, Harlan. The name originated from an Old English surname that means 'hare land'.

Imogen: Imogen likely originated from the Gaelic word, inghean, which means maiden. Shakespeare gave the princess in *Cymbeline* this name, and he based her on the character, Innogen.

Lilith: The name Lilith is derived from the Akkadian word, lilitu, which means 'of the night'. This is the same name as the demon in the ancient Assyrian myths. In the Jewish faith, she was Adam's first wife who was expelled from Eden and then replaced by Eve because Lilith was not willing to submit to him. The offspring that Lilith and Adam produced were the evil spirits.

Mavis: The name Mavis comes from Old French origin, and is the name of a bird. The bird is also referred to as a song thrush. The first 'person' that was ever given this name was one of the characters in Marie Corelli's book *The Sorrows of Satan*.

Naya: The origin of Naya comes from Arabic where it means 'new'. It is also a form of the names, Naia and Nia.

Ophelia: This name is derived from the Greek word *ophelos* which means 'help'. Jacopo Sannazaro, a 15th-century poet, is probably the one who created this name in his poem "Arcadia". Shakespeare then borrowed the name in his play "Hamlet".

Trinity: Trinity is an English name that is given in honor of Christian beliefs that God is one essence, but has three expressions: Father, Son, and Holy Spirit. Trinity only became a given name in the 20th century.

Uri: The name Uri is of Biblical and Hebrew origins. In the Old Testament, this was the name of the father, Bezalel. The meaning of the name is 'my fire or my light'.

Unisex

Ainsley: This unisex name is from Gaelic origin and began life as a Scottish surname, which was taken from the home name of Ainsley. This name was derived from element name *Ægen's* or *Æne's*, as well as the Old English *Leah*, which means 'enclosure, meadow, clearing, or wood'.

Arlo: There are many different origins for this unisex name. In Old English, it's believed to have come from the Anglo-Saxon word *here* meaning 'war, troops, fortified, and army' and the word *hlaw* meaning 'fortified hill, cairn, and mound'. From Italian origin, it is derived from the names, Karlos, Carlos, which is a variant of the English name, Charles.

August: Month names have come in and out of popularity, and August has recently hit a stride as a popular unisex name. August originates from the German form of the Latin word Augustus. It means 'to be venerable, majestic, or dignity'.

Blaine: The unisex name Blaine is believed to have Gaelic origins. In most translations, Blaine means either 'lean or thin', in certain translations it means 'yellow' or 'the source of a river'.

Bodhi: This unisex name comes from 'the tree that Buddha sat under,' which is where he gained his enlightenment. Bodhi is a Sanskrit word which means enlightenment or awakening. The Bodhi tree is a big fig tree. As opposed to some other spiritual and religious names, Bodhi has a more friendly and upbeat meaning.

Braidy: This name is a fun twist on Brady with Irish and Old English origin. The definition is a bit unclear, ranging from broad-chested to broad-eyed to a broad island. Broad is the one word that ties them all together. In Old English it came from the elements *brad* meaning 'broad' and *eage* meaning 'eye'.

Carson: This unisex name comes from Scottish and Middle English origin. It is a transferred use of a surname which means 'Carr's son'. In Scottish origin, it means 'carre', which is mossy place or marsh, and car. In Welsh, it means 'caer' which is a fort, and in Gaelic, it means 'carr' which is a rock.

Cody: Cody comes from the Gaelic surname Ó *Cuidighthigh*, which means to be a 'descendant of Cuidightheach'. Cody also has the meaning of 'helpful or pillow'.

Cohen: This unisex name is a very common Jewish surname that is believed to mean priest. As a surname, Cohen is royal name in the Jewish faith. Some may be unaware of the meaning behind the name and find it cool sounding for a first name. Some religious groups may find it offensive if used as a first name.

Dallas: While it may be a Texas City, it has origins in Scotland, meaning 'a meadow dwelling'. It is derived from the Gaelic word *dail* which means 'field' and *eas* which means 'waterfall'.

Dana: Dana comes from many different origins. One such meaning is to come from 'Dame' meaning Denmark. Dana is also another form of the name *Danu* which is a Celtic goddess of fertility. In Persia, the name means 'knowledgeable'.

Darian: The meaning of Darian is 'upholder of the good'. The name has Persian routes. Darian is a variation of Darius which is a royal Persian name.

Devon: Devon is a derivation of the Irish name Devin, which is derived from the Gaelic word *damh* which means 'a poet'. Devon means 'a defender'. It is also believed to be derived from the name of an English county, Devon. This county received its name from the Celtic tribe, Dumnonii.

Dian: Dian comes from many origins. In French, Dian means 'the divine'. In German, it comes from mythology that means 'from the God of wine.' In Indonesian, it means a 'candle'. Depending on the country and culture, Dian has several different meanings.

Emery: This unisex name was introduced to the English by the Normans and is still a rare name to hear. Emery is the Norman form of Emmerich. The name survived through the Middle Ages, and most of the modern use of it has been inspired by the surname, Emery. The name has different meanings such as 'power, universal, work, and home'.

Hadley: Hadley originated from an English surname which means 'heather field'. Hadley has always been a unisex name. Another meaning for Hadley is 'Heath near the wasteland'.

Harlow: Harlow originated from an Old English surname that had been derived from a place name known as *hœr* meaning 'rock' or the word *here* meaning 'army' which was combined with the word *hlaw* meaning 'hill'.

Haven: This unisex name originates from an English word that means 'safe place'. It ultimately came from the Old English word 'hœfen'. This is a great name for parents that don't want to go as far as heaven.

Indiana: This unisex name comes from the American state, Indiana, which means 'land of the Indians'. In England, it also means the country of India.

Indigo: This name comes from the English word indigo, which refers to the purplish-blue dye or color. The word originally was derived from the Greek word *Indikon* which means 'Indic, from India'.

Jaya: The name Jaya is derived from a Sanskrit word that means 'victory'. This came from a transcription of the feminine form of the Hindu Goddess, Durga and the masculine form of several Hindu text characters. As a modern name, in Southern India, it is used as both male and female but in the North it is more commonly female.

Jazz: Jazz is a great unisex name if you are a fan of the music, but as a name, it originated from the name Jasmine. Jasmine is a tropical plant that is commonly used in teas and perfumes.

Jersey: The meaning of this unisex name is Grassy Island. The name originated from the English culture where it originated. Jersey is a Channel Island off of the UK coast, as well as Guernsey.

Kai: The unisex name, Kai, is a Hawaiian word meaning sea. Kai in Mandarin Chinese has several meanings such as 'victory' and 'open'. In Japanese, Kai has the meaning of 'ocean, recovery, shell, and restoration'.

Lane: Lane comes from an English surname that means 'from the narrow road'. The surname originated with a person that lived close to a lane.

Marlow: This name comes from an Old English word which means driftwood. The very first phrase literally meant 'lake leavings'. It soon became a place name in Buckinghamshire, England, and then changed to a surname that was given to families that lived in that area.

Misha: There are two different meanings and origins for the name, Misha. One is Hebrew which means 'who resembles God?' The other is Russian which is the pet form of Michael.

Neo: In Africa, this unisex name means gift and in English, the name means 'new'. Neo is of Greek origin.

Orion: This unisex name comes from Greek origin meaning 'the hunter or son of fire'. In Roman and Greek mythology, Orion was Poseidon's son. He was loved by Diana, a goddess, but accidentally died at her hands. He was then placed in the heavens as the constellation.

Penn: This unisex name is of English origin, and is a more popular surname than given name. The meaning of Penn is 'enclosure or corral'.

Phoenix: This name comes from Greek and Egyptian mythology referring to a beautiful and immortal bird. After the bird lived many centuries in the Arabian Desert, the bird would be overtaken by fire and then rise out of its own ashes. This cycle would repeat every 500 years. The name derived from the Greek word *Phoinix* which means 'dark red'.

Quinn: Quinn comes from an Irish surname, which is an Anglicized version of *Ó Cuinn*, which means 'descendant of Conn'. The name was derived from the word *conn* which means 'intelligence, wisdom, or reason'.

Remy: The name Remy is a French form of Remigius, a Latin name. The Latin name was derived from the Latin word *remigis* meaning 'oarsman'.

Rowan: Rowan is a name that was derived from an Irish surname that is an Anglicized version of *Ó Ruadhain* which means 'descendant of Ruadhan'. Another origin of this name is from the rowan tree.

Sage: The name sage originated from Latin where sage refers to a plant that is seen by many to have special cleansing and healing properties. It can also refer to a person that is seen as very wise.

Shae: Shae is of Gaelic origin, and it means 'to be admirable'. It comes from the Anglicized form of the word *seaghdha*.

Storm: The name storm comes from the Old English word, storm, and it also originated from the Old Norse word *stormr*.

Val: Val comes from the name Valentine, which originated from the Roman cognomen Valentinus.

This originated from the name Valens, which means 'healthy, strong, and vigorous'.

Ziv: Ziv is a Hebrew unisex name that means 'radiant and bright'. This is the same name as the second month of the Jewish calendar.

Conclusion

Thanks for making it through to the end of *Baby Names: The Ultimate Book of Baby Names – Includes the Latest Trends, Meanings, Origins and Spiritual Significance.* Let's hope it was informative and able to provide you with all of the tools you need to achieve your goals of picking the best baby name.

The next thing is to make the hard decision of picking only one name for your little bundle of joy.

Finally, if you found this book useful in any way, a review on Amazon is always appreciated!

Made in the USA
Lexington, KY
05 April 2018